Tables of c⌐

Chapter 1

Chapter 2

Chapter 3

Chapter 4

Chapter 5

O'BRIEN Holmes

O'BRIEN Holmes

Title: Best ways to keep Fit at 40+
Sub: Strategic Guide on how to maintain your perfect Body

O'BRIEN Holmes

<u>Summary</u>

O'BRIEN Holmes

Chapter 1

7 Proven Easy ways to working out @ 40 years

HOW TO MAKE WORKING OUT FUN: Do you frequently wonder how other individuals like working out? Do you regard working out as merely one more item on your lengthy to-do list? What if you learned to link exercise with joy and anticipation instead? If you've spent much of your life disliking working out or equating exercise with suffering, it's time to modify how you think and learn how to love working out.

O'BRIEN Holmes

we're doing more and more from home - including working and working out. But many individuals find working out at home less motivating. With no one around to support you and motivate you to attain your fitness objectives, it's simpler to let working out go by the wayside. It's more crucial than ever to find how to make working out pleasurable.

Is it possible to go from disliking working out to truly loving it? The answer is yes - if you are determined to adjusting your perspective and making the adjustments required.

Like mastering any new ability, knowing how to love exercise is part mentality and part practice. By adopting the mentality that exercise is joyful, you're able to

O'BRIEN Holmes

embrace fitness as part of a comprehensive health plan. Learning how to appreciate working out becomes a tremendous tool for improving your health and attaining the physique you desire – and the wonderful life you deserve.

Aerobic exercise for weight reduction is fun, and there are numerous methods to figure out how to love working out.\s.

HOW TO ENJOY WORKING OUT: GUIDING PRINCIPLE

What are the core concepts behind learning how to appreciate working out? The U.S. Office of Disease Prevention and Health Promotion claims that there are five crucial components in appreciating exercise and making it a habit: pleasure, self-efficacy, social support,

O'BRIEN Holmes

accountability and integration into your everyday life. Since the most successful fitness regimen is one you'll stick to, the first component – learning how to love exercise – is crucial.

Building self-confidence is also vital. If you're afraid or uncertain, your anxieties will damage your attempts to exercise. Social support plays a significant part in how to enjoy working out, as people are social beings affected by their peer groups. Those peer groups promote responsibility, another crucial aspect in learning how to love working out. And by incorporating exercise into your everyday routine, it becomes a habit. From here, you're able to work out for your health and fun.

Exercise, whether to shed weight or enhance your health, may be fun. There

O'BRIEN Holmes

are methods to figure out how to start loving working out instead of hating it.

1. CHANGE YOUR BELIEFS ABOUT WORKING OUT

Want to learn how to love exercise? It all begins with assessing your thoughts and replacing negative beliefs with positive ones. Many of your views were established in childhood. If you participated in tedious P.E. courses or were compelled to be on the track team when you loathed running, you likely formed the attitude that working out was something to be endured instead than enjoyed.

Take time to explore your thoughts around exercise: Which are negative and which are positive? Where did the bad beliefs originate from? Are they still valid

in your adult life or are you clinging to outmoded notions that no longer help you? Once you recognize which ideas are limiting you from learning how to enjoy working out, you can focus on converting them into the positive thoughts that help you reach your objectives.
body fitness motivation

2. ADJUST YOUR FOCUS intensively:

Many individuals have problems learning how to enjoy working out because they are concentrated on just one outcome: weight reduction.

When you consider exercise merely as a technique to control weight, it becomes a "should" or an obligation. As Tony advises, don't "should" all over yourself! Instead of considering working exercise as a technique to lose weight, remind yourself that your body is yours to take care of and that every single choice you make – whether good or harmful – has the power to benefit or injure you.

When you start concentrating on revitalizing your body, improving your health and enriching your life, you will start to perceive exercise as a healthy option instead of an obligation. Then working exercise becomes a natural extension of taking care of oneself. This alteration in your mentality might also help you learn how to enjoy working out at home. You will no longer need the social pressure factor to urge you to work out. When you are exercising for yourself and not for others, it's lot simpler to feel motivated.

3. FIND THE RIGHT TYPE OF WORKOUT:

How to love exercise is all about selecting the correct sort of activity. Take some time and reflect back to a period when you liked physical activities. Were you with buddies, in a team or going solo? In a stunning outdoor environment? Participating in a sport? Working out does not have to entail going to a gym and jogging on a treadmill for half an hour. It might simply entail partaking in physical activities you enjoy.

Taking a karate class or rehearsing your child's cheerleading routine with them provides the same health advantages as jogging or using the elliptical machine. Many individuals skip exercise because they assume it has to appear a specific way to qualify as "working out." This simply isn't true. Any sort of physical activity that boosts your heart rate is a form of exercise. When you discover an activity that makes you joyful, you'll look forward to it instead of avoiding it. This is one of the finest things you can do while you're learning how to make working out pleasurable.

4. MAKE SURE YOU HAVE THE ENERGY TO EXERCISE:
Learning how to love working out is a rather intimidating undertaking when you barely have enough energy to do your basic daily duties. Joint discomfort and soreness may also deplete your enthusiasm and leave you asking how to make working out pleasant.

If a lack of energy or inflammation are stopping you from working out, you need to review your general lifestyle. Are you consuming fresh whole foods and rich in fiber? Are you drinking lots of water and

O'BRIEN Holmes

taking the correct supplements? Do you have effective techniques to handle stress?

Poor food, lack of self-care and a build-up of stress may sap your vitality. Working from home paired with additional child care obligations might leave you feeling fatigued and frustrated. How to love working out lowers quite low on your list of priorities when it's all you can do to simply get through the day. After a day of working from home, it's not very inspirational to merely step into the next room for your exercise.

If your lifestyle is a barrier to understanding how to appreciate exercise, accept Tony Robbins' 10-Day Challenge. You'll give yourself the gift of greater energy, a healthy diet, optimum attention and physical fitness. Once you make healthy adjustments, you'll free up the energy required to discover how to love working out.

5. CREATE TIME TO WORK OUT:

You can't learn how to appreciate exercise if you don't make the time in your schedule to work out. If you walk into your work out feeling hurried or that you are sacrificing too much of your time by working out, you aren't going to enjoy your experience.

Maybe you normally squeezed your exercise in on your way home from the office, and with remote work, your schedule has gone wild. Or maybe you've reached that winter fitness rut, when it gets dark early and all you want to do after work is go home.

O'BRIEN Holmes

Or maybe you believe that if you don't have time to exercise in the morning, you might as well not bother - but this isn't true. While morning exercises are an exhilarating way to set a wonderful tone for your day, it isn't the only time you can squeeze an effective workout in. Working exercise at any hour of the day is better than not working out at all. Oftentimes, the thought that you don't have time to exercise is only an excuse that arises from your limiting beliefs rather than a genuine scheduling constraint.

The fact is, you must make time to do the things you enjoy — and that includes working out. Don't create excuses - instead, find a solution. Set up your elliptical in front of your TV and work out as you watch your favorite comedy. Take 15-minute breaks at work and walk around the block. While your youngster is at football practice, power-walk around the field. When you understand you don't need to cut out crucial elements of your life to work out, you may learn how to enjoy working out without feeling guilty.

6. CREATE AN INSPIRING SPACE: Want to uncover how to enjoy working out at home? Your environment may have more to do with it than you believe. While many of us don't have room for a whole yoga studio in our living spaces, setting off a portion of a room or utilizing a room divider may work just as well. A basement is another wonderful choice for keeping a few items of home gym equipment. You don't need a ton of room. Just enough to make your exercise pleasant.

Music is another crucial component of learning how to love exercise. In one study, researchers examined three groups of participants: those who listened to music while exercising, those who listened to a podcast and those who listened to nothing.

Music improved satisfaction by 28% compared to those with no auditory stimulation and by 13% compared to those who listened to a podcast. Researchers found that since music evoked a more pleasant emotional state during exercise, music is a wonderful tool for learning how to enjoy working out – and you can utilize it whether your training area is in your house or in the vast outdoors.

O'BRIEN Holmes

7. LEARN TO BE MORE ADAPTABLE:

Humans seek predictability, even in our workout regimens. We're also incredibly sociable people, hard-wired to work together and enjoy gatherings. When it comes to learning how to make working out pleasurable, there is power in numbers. One research indicated that our social networks impact our exercise-related behaviour. Participants who spent time with healthy companions were more likely to effectively reduce weight and enjoy exercise than those whose peers were not oriented toward healthier living.

If you're having problems learning how to enjoy working out at home without your social network, move your attention to build a growth mindset that will motivate you to master new things.

O'BRIEN Holmes

In addition to adjusting your thinking, mix up your routine, too. Variety is also one of our core human needs, so alter up your fitness program each week to avoid from becoming bored. Join a digital fitness challenge or an online community where you may obtain encouragement. Connecting with other individuals in similar circumstances is a terrific approach to recall how to appreciate working out. Remember what Tony says: "Every challenge is a gift — without troubles we would not grow." How can you utilize your present obstacles to achieve progress in your life?

Chapter 2

DIFFICULTY IN LOSING WEIGHT AT
40+ AND STAYING POSITIVE:

Yes!!! Fitness is for life. Motivate yourself
with these practical tips.

Have you ever started a fitness program
and then quit? If you answered yes,
you're not alone. Many people start
fitness programs, but they may stop
when they get bored, they don't enjoy it
or results come too slowly. Here are
seven tips to help you stay motivated.

1. Set goals:
Start with simple goals and then progress
to longer range goals. Remember to make
your goals realistic and achievable. It's
easy to get frustrated and give up if your
goals are too ambitious.

O'BRIEN Holmes

For example, if you haven't exercised in a while, a short-term goal might be to walk 10 minutes a day five days a week. Even short amounts of exercise can have benefits. An intermediate goal might be to walk 30 minutes five days a week. A long-term goal might be to complete a 5K walk.

For most healthy adults, the Department of Health and Human Services recommends at least 150 minutes of moderate aerobic activity or 75 minutes of vigorous aerobic activity a week, or a combination of moderate and vigorous activity. Greater amounts of exercise will provide even greater benefit. Aim to incorporate strength training exercises of all the major muscle groups into your fitness routine at least two times a week.

2. Make it fun:
Find sports or activities that you enjoy, then vary the routine to keep it interesting. If you're not enjoying your workouts, try something different. Join a volleyball or softball league. Take a ballroom dancing class. Check out a health club or martial arts center. If you like to work out at home, look online for videos of many types of exercise classes, such as yoga, high-intensity interval training or kickboxing. Or take a walk or jog in a local park. Discover your hidden athletic talent or interests.

Remember, exercise doesn't have to be boring, and you're more likely to stick with a fitness program if you're having fun.

3. Make physical activity part of your daily routine:

O'BRIEN Holmes

If it's hard to find time for exercise, don't fall back on excuses. Schedule workouts as you would any other important activity.

You can also slip in physical activity throughout the day. Take the stairs instead of the elevator, or park further away from the store. Walk up and down sidelines while watching the kids play sports. Take a walk during a break at work.

If you work from home, stretch, walk or climb your stairs on breaks. Or do squats, lunges or situps. Walk your dog if you have one. Pedal a stationary bike, walk or jog on a treadmill, or do strength training exercises during your lunch break or while you watch TV at night.

Research has found that sitting for long periods of time may negatively affect your health, even if you otherwise get the recommended amount of weekly activity. If you sit for several hours a day at work, aim to take regular breaks during the day to move, such as walking to get a drink of water or standing during phone conversations or video meetings.

4. Put it on paper:

Are you hoping to lose weight? Boost your energy? Sleep better? Manage a chronic condition? Write down your goals. Seeing the benefits of regular exercise and writing your goals down on paper may help you stay motivated.

You may also find that it helps to keep an exercise diary. Record what you did during each exercise session, how long you exercised and how you felt afterward.

O'BRIEN Holmes

Recording your efforts and tracking your progress can help you work toward your goals and remind you that you're making progress.

5. Join forces with friends, neighbors or others:
You're not in this alone. Invite friends or co-workers to join you when you exercise or go on walks. Work out with your partner or other loved ones. Play soccer with your kids. Organize a group of neighbors to take fitness classes at a local health club or work out together virtually on video.

6. Reward yourself:
After each exercise session, take a few minutes to savor the good feelings that exercise gives you. This type of internal reward can help you make a long-term commitment to regular exercise.

O'BRIEN Holmes

External rewards can help too. When you reach a longer range goal, treat yourself to a new pair of walking shoes or new tunes to enjoy while you exercise.

7. Be flexible:

If you're too busy to work out or simply don't feel up to it, take a day or two off. Go easy on yourself if you need a break. The important thing is to get back on track as soon as you can.

Now that you've regained your enthusiasm, get moving! Set your goals, make it fun and pat yourself on the back from time to time. Remember, physical activity is for life. Review these tips whenever you feel your motivation slipping.

Why Is It So Hard To Lose Weight After 40?

It is not a secret that losing weight becomes more difficult with age. People who easily shed some pounds in their youth feel helpless and desperate when they can't lose their weight as they get older. But why is it so hard to lose weight after 40? The main reasons are (3):

Age-Related Muscle Loss:
As you age, the amount of lean muscles in your body decreases. This process is called sarcopenia (8). You may also lose muscles if you suffer from arthritis or a certain injury, and thus move less. Since your muscle mass decreases, your body burns fewer calories, which then makes it more difficult to slim down using the same methods you used to.

Hormonal Changes:
Men and women all go through hormonal changes as they age. Oftentimes these changes lead to weight gain. When men hit 40 their testosterone levels start to gradually decrease. This hormone, among other things, regulates fat distribution and muscle mass. This means its reduction makes your body burn fewer calories.

Another factor that makes it more difficult to shed pounds after 40 is a decrease in the production of growth hormone. This is responsible for many processes, including the growth and maintenance of muscle mass. So, its decrease also reduces the number of calories your body burns.

Decrease In Physical Activity:
As you become older, you tend to move less. Vigorous physical activity may take too much energy and effort, and sometimes even cause pain or certain health problems. This makes it very difficult to burn the extra calories which your diet doesn't reduce.

40-Year-Old Male Diet Plan Basics
If all your life you have been leading a healthy lifestyle, then you shouldn't worry about weight gain after 40. Perhaps, you will need to make some slight changes in your routine, but nothing drastic. However, if you like to munch on fast food every now and then, spend the first half of your day in a chair, and the second half on the couch or in bed, and every evening you enjoy a glass

of wine or a bottle of beer, then your weight loss is almost inevitable. Luckily, it is never too late to get on the right path and start leading a healthy lifestyle. If you are wondering: "What is the best way for a man to lose weight?", "How to lose weight fast for men?", or even "How to lose weight when you're over 55?", then we have got exactly what you need. Here are the 40-year-old male diet plan basics to help you achieve and maintain your desired weight (2):

Count Your Calories:

No matter what age you are, if your goal is to stay toned, you need to make sure that you burn all the calories that you consume. If you dream of slimming down, then calorie restriction is your go-to. To successfully shed some pounds, you need to reduce your caloric intake so that you eat less than you burn (10).

Now, you want to make sure that you don't cut your energy intake too drastically. Experts recommend reducing your daily caloric intake by 500-1,000 calories. Such a move will result in a loss of 1-2 pounds (0.45-1kg) of fat a week (4). And if you don't need to shed pounds, but would rather maintain your current weight, then use a calculator to find out how many calories your body requires, and make sure that you don't consume more.

Chapter 3

THE MASTERS GUIDE ON GETTING BACK TO SHAPE AT 40+:
Exercises for Men Over 40 to Get Back Into Shape...

Men should generally Protect their health and maintain in shape, especially when you're older.

Men older than 40 may lose 8 percent or more of their muscular mass every 10 years. Getting back into shape might seem like a major job if you've been idle or exercise infrequently. You can do it if you are willing to put in the time and effort. The best fitness regimen for guys older than 40 involves strength training, flexibility exercises, and aerobic activity.

O'BRIEN Holmes

Before beginning any workout plan, consult your healthcare practitioner.

Strength Training: Strength training is necessary to help avoid loss of muscle mass and to increase physical strength. A strength-training strategy to get back into shape after age 40 should include routines for all muscle groups. Rotate training your muscles on a plan with a day of rest between exercising muscle groups. Dumbbells, barbells, and resistance workout machine routines may enable you to grow a leaner, stronger body. Body-weight exercises, such squats, crunches, and plank motions, should be added into your strength-training routine. Start carefully by completing eight to 10 repetitions of strength exercises. Increase the weight or repetitions as you build strength.

Cardio: \sCardiovascular, or aerobic, exercise is a crucial part of every fitness strategy. Cardio exercises enhance your heart rate and respiration. You burn fat while you are increasing muscle and endurance. Try to obtain at least 30 minutes of moderate aerobic exercise per day. Swimming, walking, jogging, and running are good aerobic exercises. Gym activities for cardio include riding a stationary bicycle and operating a treadmill, stair-step, or elliptical machine.

Flexibility: \sStretching workouts enhance your joint flexibility and range of motion. Stretching your muscles after warming up could minimize your probability of muscle strain or joint injury. Stretching also prepares your muscles for more difficult exercise, such as weightlifting or resistance band activities, for higher sports performance. Stretch your muscles after an exercise session to aid calm down your body and begin the muscular tissue repair process after intense exertion.

Warm Up and Cool Down: \sWarm up before exercising to help prepare your body for more rigorous activities. Warming up gradually boosts your heart rate and improves blood flow to all parts of your body. Warm-up routines may aid lessen the likelihood of muscle tension or a sprained joint. Warm up for strength training by going through the acts of lifting weights without the weights. If you wish to run, walk briskly for roughly five minutes before initiating your run. Cool down by completing your exercise routine at a slower tempo for the last 10 minutes of your workout. Runners may cool down by walking for 10 minutes.

Chapter 4

Diet for rapid weight loss at 40+ years :

This is one of the most extensive posts on this site (and one we update every year) because we want to hand you the proven 5 step guide to lose weight — and keep it off — as a man over 40.

If you don't have 10 minutes to carefully read this article right now, bookmark this page and come back later. You won't want to miss a thing!

If you diligently read this article and understand this five-step process, you will have the big picture plan of weight loss for men over 40.

"I'll just cut my carbs, scale back my portions, and start exercising again ... I'm bound to drop some weight!"

Have you heard anything like that before? Or even said it yourself?

This "shotgun" weight loss approach sounds simple enough, and it's the general plan that most guys over 40 follow when trying to lose weight.

The BIG problem is that 92% of men fail at sustaining weight loss by using this general approach (according to data from the University of Scranton).

Tens of millions of guys (probably yourself included) are failing on diets because they are not following a specialized plan that integrates the five necessary steps of weight loss for men over 40.

Any unspecific or "cookie-cutter" weight loss plan won't work for you long-term as a guy in your 40s, 50s, or 60s.

Your body is undergoing a whole slew of metabolic and hormonal changes that need to be accounted for to lose weight effectively.

Instead of failing at weight loss again (and again), here's what you need to start doing instead ...

Step 1: DO NOT Start With Diet and Exercise

O'BRIEN Holmes

One of the biggest mistakes guys make when trying to lose weight is that they attack diet and exercise first.

This is a SUPER EASY mistake to make because it seems like diet and exercise would be the "perfect" place to start when trying to lose weight.

Yet, this is the WRONG first step.

Although both diet and exercise are very important (we'll discuss those extensively in Steps 3-5), there are two prior foundations that you need to build first.

Foundation 1: Sleep Optimization For Weight Loss
Foundation 2:

The Proper Weight Loss Success Mindset

Poor Sleep Forces Your Body To Rampantly Store Fat EVEN IF You Are Following A Good Nutrition Plan
During sleep, your body regulates all of its major weight loss hormones.

Your body absolutely requires balanced levels of these hormones to lose weight effectively.

Weight loss for men over 40 is dramatically impacted because of these hormone levels.

Here are the most prominent hormones that impact your weight loss...

Growth hormone — a key anti-aging hormone — naturally surges at night to help your body burn fat, build muscle, & repair tissues.
Insulin — a key food and fat storage hormone — decreases to its lowest levels

at night, enabling your metabolism to burn a ton of fat.

Cortisol — your body's main stress hormone — decreases at night allowing your cells to relax and rejuvenate. Without proper sleep, these critical fat-burning and fat-storing hormones get ALL sorts of messed up — literally forcing your body to hold onto fat.

In fact, after a single night of disrupted sleep, your body experiences lower growth hormone, higher cortisol, a slower metabolic rate, and greater insulin resistance.

How effective do you think your weight loss efforts will be as you're pushing against this terrible hormonal cascade?

Your weight loss progress will flat out suck if you're not getting enough sleep.

O'BRIEN Holmes

In fact, a study from the University of Chicago showed that people trying to lose weight with inadequate sleep experienced profound MUSCLE LOSS — with little to no fat loss.

That's the exact opposite of the result you want.

Adequate sleep is the foundation of your weight loss success — you should be getting a MINIMUM of 6-7 hours a night. goal.

Anyone who says differently is either full of crap or hasn't been through the process themselves!

Transforming your health and body requires unwinding the unhealthy lifestyle habits that got you overweight in the first place.

O'BRIEN Holmes

This means your eating patterns, habits for coping with stress, exercise habits (or lack thereof), and more.

We need to shift you AWAY from the bad habits that are keeping you stuck, while also moving TOWARDS the new healthy habits that will support your goals.

As you can imagine, this degree of health change takes effort.

That's precisely why your successful and sustainable weight loss requires you to develop a strong mindset with the emotional fortitude to handle making these healthy changes over the long term.

Speaking of mindset, check out how this Fit Father used a military mindset to lose 43 lbs in less than three months.

O'BRIEN Holmes

You need to develop a mindset that is
DEEPLY and FULLY committed to your
weight loss journey.

How do we find motivation for weight
loss, working out, or sticking to a healthy
diet?

We either push our way through with
"willpower," or we find our "why-power"
to push us through.

It may be to stay strong to take care of
your spouse.

I've found (in most cases) the strongest
"Why Powers" are almost always rooted
in something bigger than you as
individuals.

Take a minute now to think about your
weight loss "WHY"Very low-calorie diet;
VLCD; Low-calorie diet; LCD; Very low

energy diet; Weight loss – fast weight reduction; Overweight - fast weight reduction; Obesity - fast weight loss; Diet - fast weight reduction; Intermittent fasting - quick weight reduction; Time-restricted eating - fast weight reduction

A rapid weight loss diet is a sort of diet in which you lose more than 2 pounds (1 kilogram, kg) a week over many weeks. To lose weight thus rapidly you consume extremely few calories.

How It Works?

O'BRIEN Holmes

These diets are most typically adopted by persons with obesity who wish to reduce weight rapidly. These diets are less typically suggested by health care practitioners. People on these diets should be observed regularly by a provider. Rapid weight reduction may not be safe for some individuals to achieve on their own.

These diets are intended to be taken for a limited period and are typically not suggested for more than a few weeks. The forms of quick weight reduction diets are mentioned below.

Persons who lose weight extremely rapidly are far more likely to regain the weight over time than people who lose weight slowly via less dramatic food modifications and physical exercise. Weight reduction is a higher stress for the body, and the hormonal reaction to the weight loss is considerably stronger. The hormonal reaction is one of the reasons why weight reduction slows down over time and also why weight gain happens when the diet is interrupted or relaxed.

Very Low-Calorie Diet (VLCD): \sOn a VLCD, you may consume as little as 800 calories a day and may lose up to 3 to 5 pounds (1.5 to 2 kg) per week. Most VLCDs employ meal substitutes, such as formulae, soups, shakes, and bars instead of normal meals. This helps ensure that you obtain all of the nutrients you need each day.

A VLCD is only suggested for individuals who have obesity and need to reduce weight for health reasons. These diets are typically used before weight-loss surgery. You should only utilize a VLCD with the aid of your physician. Most experts do not advocate adopting a VLCD for more than 12 weeks.

Low-Calorie Diet (LCD): \ These diets normally allow roughly 1,000 to 1,200 calories a day for women and 1,200 to 1,600 calories a day for males. An LCD is a better option than a VLCD for most individuals who wish to lose weight rapidly. But you should still be overseen by a provider. You will not lose weight as quickly with an LCD, but you can lose just as much weight with a VLCD. Time-Restricted Eating:\sThis diet method is getting increasingly popular. It is frequently likened to fasting, however, the two techniques are somewhat different. Time-restricted eating restricts the number of hours per day that you may eat. A prominent technique is 16:8. For this plan, you have to eat all of your meals throughout 8 hours, for example, 10 am to 6 pm. The remainder of the time you cannot eat anything. There is some research suggesting this strategy may promote quick weight reduction, but there is little evidence so far concerning whether the weight loss is maintained.

Chapter 5

8 Ways to Think Thin Mentally:

Motivation to reduce weight frequently reaches an all-time high when the first buds of spring break up, signifying that bathing suit season is not long behind. And although there's no getting past the need to exercise and eat properly, long-term weight reduction begins in your thinking. Experts suggest that having the appropriate mentality might help you imagine yourself as skinny.

If you want to succeed at weight reduction, you need to "reduce the mental fat, and that will lead to reducing the waistline fat," says Pamela Peeke, MD, author of Fit to Live. "Look at the patterns and behaviors in your life that you are carrying about with you that get in the way of achievement."

Everyone has their justifications. When attempting to change their lifestyle and nutrition, most individuals do OK until something occurs — whether it's job pressure, family troubles, or something else. Whatever your particular difficulty, the pattern has to alter if you want to be successful.

O'BRIEN Holmes

"I want to enable individuals to recognize these patterns, deal with the true causes, so they can go on and be able to succeed at healing their health," adds Peeke.

Dieting doesn't mean you can't munch. Take this quiz for sensible eating suggestions.

To Think Yourself Thin, Have Patience One key mental impediment to weight reduction is desiring too much, too soon. Blame it on our quick-gratification culture, with its instant texting, PDAs, and digital cameras: Weight reduction is too gradual to please most dieters.

"Losers seek instant results. ... Even though it took them years to acquire weight, once they start to lose weight, they have little patience with the suggested 1-2 pounds each week," says

O'BRIEN Holmes

Cynthia Sass, MS, RD, a representative for the American Dietetic Association.

But you'll receive the finest outcomes when you lose weight slowly. Sass tells her customers that when they lose weight too rapidly, they're frequently shedding mainly water or lean tissue, not fat.

"When you lose lean tissue, metabolism slows down, making it much tougher to lose weight," she says.

Think Thin: 8 Strategies
Get that overweight attitude out of your brain and start thinking like a skinny person with these eight strategies:

1. Picture Yourself Thin:
If you want to be skinny, envision yourself thin. Visualize your future self,

six months to a year down the line, and think about how amazing you'll look and feel without the excess pounds. Dig out old images of your slimmer self and put them in a spot as a reminder of what you are aiming for. Ask yourself what you did back then that you could put into your lifestyle now. And, suggests Peeke, think about things you would want to undertake but can't due to your weight.

"To overcome old patterns, you need to perceive oneself favorably," Peeke explains.

2. Have Realistic Expectations:
When physicians ask their patients how much they want to weigh, the amount is frequently reasonably feasible. Peeke has her patients pick a realistic weight range, not a single figure.

"I ask them to think forward 12 months, and would they be happy being 12 or 24 pounds thinner?" she adds "It just amounts to 1-2 pounds each month, which is achievable, sustainable, and reasonable in the context of job and family." She proposes reevaluating your weight goal after six months.

3. Set Small Goals:
Make a list of minor objectives that will help you attain your weight reduction goals.
These mini-goals should be something that will enhance your lifestyle without wrecking devastation in your life, such as:

Eating more fruits and veggies every day.
Getting some type of physical exercise for at least 30 minutes a day.
Drinking booze solely on the weekends.

O'BRIEN Holmes

Eating low-fat popcorn instead of chips,
Ordering a side salad instead of french
fries.
Being able to go up a flight of stairs
without gasping for breath.
"We all know that change is hard and it is
tougher if you attempt to make too many
changes, so start small and gradually
create lifestyle adjustments,"
recommends Sass.

4. Get Support:
We all need help, particularly during
terrible times. Find a friend, family
member, or support group you can
connect with regularly. Studies reveal
individuals who are connected with
others, whether it's in person or online,
fare better than dieters who attempt to
do it alone.

5. Create a Detailed Action Plan:

Sass proposes that each night, you plan your nutritious meals and workout for the following day. Planning is 80% of the fight. If you're prepared with a comprehensive strategy, success will follow.

"Schedule your workout as you would an appointment," Sass adds. "Pack some dried fruits, vegetables, or meal replacement snacks so you won't be tempted to consume the incorrect sorts of things."

Make your health a priority by implementing such actions into your daily, and eventually, these healthy activities will become a normal part of your existence.

6. Reward Yourself:
Pat yourself on the back with a trip to the movies, a manicure, or anything that will

O'BRIEN Holmes

help you feel good about your successes (other than food rewards) (other than food rewards).

"Reward yourself once you have reached one of your mini-goals or dropped 5 pounds or a few inches around your waist, so you acknowledge your hard work and appreciate the measures you are doing to be healthy," Peeke adds.

7. Ditch Old Habits:
Old habits die hard, but you can't continue to do things the way you used to if you want to succeed at weight reduction.

"Slowly but surely, attempt to recognize where you are participating in habits that contribute to weight gain and turn them around with modest steps that you can

easily do without feeling deprived,"
advises Sass.

For example, if you are an evening couch
potato, start by changing your snack
from a bag of cookies or chips to a piece
of fruit. The following night, try having
only a calorie-free drink. Eventually, you
can start completing activities while you
watch television.

Another method to get started
abandoning your poor habits: Get rid of
the tempting, empty-calorie meals in
your kitchen and replace them with
healthier ones.

8. Keep Track:

Weigh in often and maintain notebooks
describing what you eat, how much you
exercise, your emotions, and your weight
and measurements. Studies demonstrate

that keeping track of this information helps encourage beneficial habits and diminish negative ones. Simply knowing that you're monitoring your food consumption might help you avoid that slice of cake!

"Journals are a sort of accountability ... that assist to indicate which techniques are succeeding" explains Peeke. "When you are responsible, you are less likely to suffer food disassociations, or be 'asleep at the meal.'"

Printed in Dunstable, United Kingdom